Eliminate Acne

Top Acne Free Tricks Revealed!

By: Heather Rose

Table of Contents

PUBLISHERS NOTES

DEDICATION

This book is dedicated to individuals who suffer from acne especially during their adolescent years.

CHAPTER 1- THE TRUTH ABOUT ACNE

There are so many misconceptions about what exactly causes acne and why certain people suffer from it while others live a blemish-free life, never having to experience the pain from excessive acne.

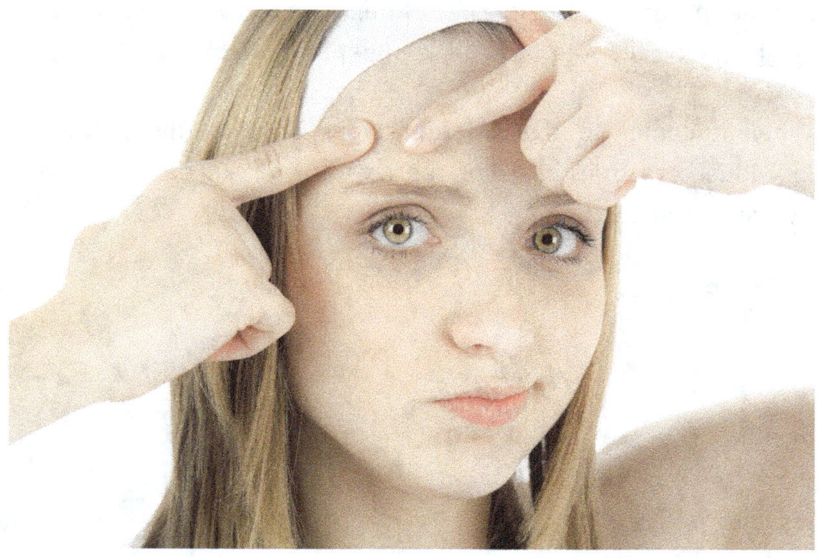

With these myths and ridiculous notions comes another set of problems. People suffering from acne are so desperate to eliminate it, that they try all sorts of different approaches, from modifying their diet, to over-tanning believing that it will minimize acne permanently.

These methods can end up being detrimental to your attempts at controlling your acne, and in many cases can actually intensify your acne and cause it to get worse. In some cases, these 'instant cure remedies' can end up causing permanent scarring.

So, what is acne really all about?

For starters, regardless of what you've heard, acne is not life threatening and no one has ever died from acne itself. By clinical terms, acne is described as being caused by a hormonal imbalance, clinically coined as 'chronic inflammation', or 'systemic inflammation'.

With chronic inflammation, the primary culprit is poor digestion, accompanied by a poor diet.

Another primary cause of acne is when pores on your body become clogged, typically your face, neck, upper body, back and even chest.

When it comes to the different types of acne, there are five individual categories based on the severity and skin damage caused by acne, including:

Comedos

Papule

Pustule

Nodule

Cyst

Symptoms of acne such as blackheads and whiteheads belong to the comedos category, with cysts being classified as belonging to the nodule category.

Another word for acne is "Acne Vulgaris", a form of acne, which commonly occurs during puberty.

It primarily affects the back, face and chest. Acne vulgaris affect both teenage boys and girls. Nearly 30-40% of teenage boys are affected between the ages of 18 and 19 years old. Girls are generally affected between the ages of 16-18 years.

Here is how acne is characterized by certain groups that can determine the severity of your acne:

Black Heads

You will suffer from black heads when your pores are partially blocked which allows some the bacteria, dead skin cells and sebum to escape and drain to the surface of your skin.

The dark color that comes with black heads is not dirt and so consistently washing your face will not prevent black heads from appearing. Black heads are firmer and often take a few days to a week to clear.

White Heads

You will see white heads appear when a pore is completely blocked, the opposite of a black head.

 With white heads, they tend to last for only a short length of time and result from sebum, bacteria and dead skin cells being trapped beneath the skins surface.

Papules

These are painful, red bumps that are inflamed and contain no head.

Pustules

A pustule is what we commonly call a "pimple". They are very similar to a white head but are always inflamed and contain a white or yellow center.

Nodules

Nodules are larger spots that can lasts for months and be difficult to deal with because of how painful they can be. Nodules are hardened bumps beneath the skins surface and with nodules, scarring is quite common.

If you believe that you have nodules, please do not squeeze them as doing so may cause severe trauma to your skin, spreading of nodules, and prolonged life.

Don't try to treat nodules on your own, instead book an appointment with your dermatologist for assistance as nodules are quite difficult to control with over the counter medications or home based remedies.

Cysts

Just like a nodule, cysts can be large and feel hard, in fact, some cysts feel like round balls within the skin.

They are also very painful and are filled with liquid. Do not squeeze or attempt to break a cyst, as you can push the bacteria and infection deeper into your skin.

Apart from the common forms of acne that many of us have experienced from time to time throughout our life, there are four types of acne that are considered more severe and should be treated by a doctor.

Acne Conglobata

This is the most severe form of acne, generally characterized by the large appearance of numerous nodules, often connected, interconnected and contains a large number of black heads. Because these lesions can become ulcerated, they can cause disfiguring and severe scarring on the skin surface.

Conglobata is usually found on the face, back, chest, upper arms and thighs.

Acne Conglobata usually affects people between the ages of 18 and 30 and is more common in males.

It should also be noted that Acne Conglobata could stay active for many years, lying dormant until something occurs that causes the acne to resurface. The cause of Acne Conglobata is unknown at this time.

Acne Fulminans

This type of severe acne is actually an abrupt onset of acne conglobata that typically afflicts young men.

The symptoms of the severe nodulocystic, often ulcerating acne, are readily apparent. As with normal cases of acne conglobata the lesions cover large portions of the extremities and the facial region, including the disfiguring scars that can eventually develop.

Yet what makes acne fulminans unique in that it also includes fever symptoms, aching of the joints, particularly the knees and hips, and varying degrees of weight loss that depend upon the individual.

Gram Negative Folliculitis

Gram-negative folliculitis is a form of extreme acne caused by an inflammation of the follicles that is caused by bacterial infection:

This condition is characterized by pustules and cysts.

It has been determined in some cases that its development is caused by a complication resulting from a long-term antibiotic treatment of acne vulgaris.

The reason that this form of acne is called "gram-negative" relates to the fact that gram is a type of blue stain used for laboratory testing for microscopic organism. Bacteria that do not stain blue are referred to as "gram-negative."

Like other forms of extreme or severe acne, gram-negative folliculitis is a rare condition, and we do not know whether it is more common in males or females as it has been documented in both.

Pyoderma Faciale

This type of severe acne affects only females, usually between the ages of 20 to 40 years of age.

It is characterized by large painful nodules, pustules and sores that may leave scarring.

Forming abruptly, pyoderma faciale may occur on the skin of a woman who has never had acne before.

Generally, this type of extreme acne is confined to the face, and though it does not last longer than a year, it can cause a great deal of damage in a very short time.

Keloidalis is a scar-like acne that can become present in both male and females, however is most prevalent among men.

Keloidalis commonly affects the neck area. When the inflamed papules and pustules grow into larger cysts and nodules, the skin gets very greasy leading to atrophic scars and keloids on the neck, shoulders and upper back.

Other types of acne include:

*Acne Rosacea - Most common in the elderly and is characterized by red rashes on the chin, nose, cheek and forehead.

*Acne Conglobata - This is a highly inflammatory disease with comedones, nodules, abscesses, and draining sinus tracts.

*Acne Fulminans - is a severe form of the skin disease, acne, which can occur after unsuccessful treatment for another form of acne such as acne conglobata.

Acne usually occurs during the teenage years of a person's life, however, adults are not immune to acne, and many of us, who fail to treat it can end up suffering from it our entire lives.

Many of the problems facing those who are trying to deal with acne are the pervasive sources of misinformation out there regarding the causes of acne.

With these myths and ridiculous notions comes another set of problems. People suffering from acne are so desperate to eliminate it, that they try all sorts of different approaches, from modifying their diet, to over-tanning believing that it will minimize acne permanently.

These methods can end up being detrimental to your attempts at controlling your acne, and in many cases can actually intensify your acne and cause it to get worse. In some cases, these 'instant cure remedies' can end up causing permanent scarring.

Rather than finding solutions and treatments to alleviate the symptoms, problems are often compounded. Ill-advised treatments based off these myths can have less than effective results and can often do further damage in the case of severe acne.

In light of the influence that these myths can have on both understanding acne in general and the courses of treatment in particular, it wodule be wise to start with a quick overview of some of the more common myths that are out there, dispelling the misinformation with the truth about them.

Chapter 2- 7 Myths About Acne

Myth #1: Acne Is Caused By Poor Hygiene

It doesn't matter how often, how ritually, you scrub your face and other areas affected by acne; this has no bearing on either the status of current a breakout or the creation of new problems. In fact, this sort of rigorous regimen of washing and scrubbing can actually irritate skin and make the acne worse, not better.

Though you may have heard so from well-meaning parents growing up or some other misinformed person, acne is not caused by poor hygiene.

This doesn't mean that hygiene isn't important. In fact, good hygiene can help reduce the effects of acne if used in conjunction with acne treatment products.

Rather than frequent, harsh washing, it is generally recommended that you wash your face twice to three times a day with mild soap and then pat it dry - don't scrub dry.

Myth #2: Acne Is Caused By Your Diet

"Don't eat chocolate, it will give you pimples!" "They say that eating greasy foods can give you zits."

Most of you have heard these and other similar statements before, right?

What they are saying, in effect, is that what you eat can cause acne. But, what they are saying isn't true. It is a myth, one of the more popular ones actually, about the causes of acne.

Extensive scientific research has been conducted, searching for possible correlations between one's diet and a possible cause of acne, and have not found anything conclusive.

However, each of us is different. Some people notice that breakouts are worse after eating certain foods--and the kinds of food differ with each person.

For example, some people may notice breakouts after eating chocolate; while others have no effects with chocolate. Instead, they notice breakouts occurring after they drink too much coffee or caffeine.

These are just examples but they might be worth heading. If there is some sort of food or drink that might be affecting your acne, then cut back and see if that helps.

Myth #3: Acne Is Caused By Stress & Anxiety

Stress is not a direct cause of acne but it is true that some types of stress can cause the body to produce a hormone called cortisol, which can irritate existing acne. Indirectly, some medication that we take to alleviate or control extreme stress or emotional problems like depression can be factors in the production of acne.

In fact, some medicines have acne listed as a possible side effect.

Myth #4: Acne Will Disappear On Its Own

This is generally not true and acne needs treatment in order to be cleared up.

With the selection of acne treatment products available today there is no reason not to investigate and find what has the best results for those concerned. In some cases, a dermatologist should be consulted and other forms of treatment can be pursued.

Myth #5: Tanning Will Eliminate Acne

In fact, this has the reverse effect.

At first it may seem that the latest bake in the tanning bed or sunbathing has improved your complexion, but in fact the tan may only have masked or covered the acne. In reality, the sun can make the skin dry and irritated and this can lead to more breakouts.

On another note, if you do tan, make sure that you are using a sunscreen that doesn't contain oils and other chemicals that might clog up your pores and cause acne to get worse. (Look for noncomedogenic or nonacnegenic on the label.)

Myth #6: Breaking The Zit Will Clear It Up

Again, though this seems true, it is another myth.

Rather than speeding up the process of healing, this action actually prolongs the situation as popping the whitehead caused the bacteria inside to be pushed deeper into the skin, which allows more infection to grow, and ultimately leads to scarring.

Myth #7: Only Teenagers Suffer From Acne

The truth is that about 25% to 30% of all people between the ages 25- 44 have active acne. So the idea that acne is only a problem for teens is yet another myth.

After covering these myths, it is important to note, that these are not all of the myths that are out there, circulating in the

Chapter 3- Reasons Why You Have Acne

Natural, holistic or at-home remedies can be an inexpensive way to combat acne.

Natural and herbal remedies

Despite extensive research into the causes of acne and why certain people consistently suffer, while others never experience a single bout of acne, it has never been scientifically proven as to the exact cause of acne.

There are however, contributing factors often associated with those who have acne and those who don't, including:

Puberty

Teenagers and zits, they always seem to go hand in hand, and it's a time in our life that even those of us who have never suffered from acne before (or after) experienced the symptoms of breakouts.

In fact, studies have revealed that over 94% of the entire population between the ages of 12 and 24 have suffered from acne at one time or another.

The reason why acne is so common amongst teenagers is based around the hormone, androgens, which begin to work overtime as we approach puberty.

Androgens can cause our hair follicles and skin pores to become enlarged and extremely oily and when the oil mixes with our skin cells, it can cause our pores to become blocked, resulting in temporary acne breakouts.

Your Hormones

Hormones seem to play a major role in causing acne, and has been consistently linked to causing severe acne in both teenagers and adults.

It's a Family Thing

It's been said that while acne is not directly hereditary, if your parents suffered from severe acne, you are far more prone to acne yourself.

Scientists are still studying the links between children with acne and parents and no concrete evidence of a direct connection is available at this time.

Your Prescriptions

Depending on the type of medication you are on, specific prescription drugs are known to cause acne to flare up, especially anti-depressant and anti-anxiety medications, as well as specific types of steroids, barbiturates and lithium.

If you are on any medication and you believe that it is causing your acne to flare up, contact your doctor and discuss alternative prescription based options that you can take to avoid causing your acne to get worse.

DO NOT stop taking your medication until you consult with your family doctor.

Our Environment

If you've been exposed to chemicals at your workplace, or even at home with household cleaners, air fresheners or scented detergents, you might find that your existing acne may become temporarily irritated.

There have also been case studies performed where people who had no former history of acne began to experience extreme breakouts after being subjected to ongoing chemical cleaners, especially when cleaning without protecting their hands with gloves.

CHAPTER 4- NATURAL ACNE REMEDIES

Natural, holistic or at-home remedies can be an inexpensive way to combat acne.

Natural and herbal remedies are derived from living plant life. If you every have taken a vitamin supplement you might have noticed the taste just before swallowing, it tastes like ground plants, leaves etc, that is because it is. There are no chemicals involved.

Natural herbal remedies do not alter hormone balance, change chemical levels in the brain or trick your body.

Why? Because the herbs contain certain properties that are meant to regulate functions the body to promote healing and health.

They are not synthetic or man-made, they are simply from the earth and are here to help with problems that we face. Herbal supplements are a healthy alternative to prescription drugs.

Some of the natural remedies are listed below.

*Drinks rich in antioxidants and Vitamin C and/or E can assist in freshening and rejuvenated skin.

*Vitamin E rich foods can diminish acne-related scarring.

*Tea tree oil is a popular home remedy for acne. It is an essential oil that is diluted and applied topically to acne lesions. Because tea tree oil can kill bacteria, applying topical tea tree oil to acne lesions is believed to kill the bacteria that cause acne.

Additionally, there are certain herbs that can be digested that can relieve chronic inflammatory problems especially relating to the skin, such as acne.

These herbs include burdock, cleavers, red clover, figwort, poke root, echinacea, and blue flag. A great combination is blue flag, burdock, yellow dock, and echinacea. These can be mixed together and infused with hot water to make a tea.

Drink a cup of this 3 times a day. You can put a little honey in it to make it taste better.

When you are investigating the over the counter options, always focus on medicine or ointments contains Benzoyl peroxide 5 percent.

Apply this to your problem areas before bed, each day.

The Benzoyl helps with open sores and pimples as well as unblocking blackheads and removes the bacteria that commonly inhabit the pores in your skin. You should only need a small amount, just a fingertip measure will do.

Benzoyl peroxide effectively kills bacteria, drys your skin and promotes the renewed growth of new cells.

You can purchase lower doses over the counter however stronger forms will require a prescription.

Here are a few of my favorite home-based remedies for instantly treating acne:

Hot And Cold Compress Packs

This is one of the most popular home based remedies and a very simple one to try. All you do is wet a towel and press it up against the area of your body that has acne, whether it's your face, chest or back.

This will reduce swelling and instantly eliminated clogged pores, which is a primary culprit in the cause of acne.

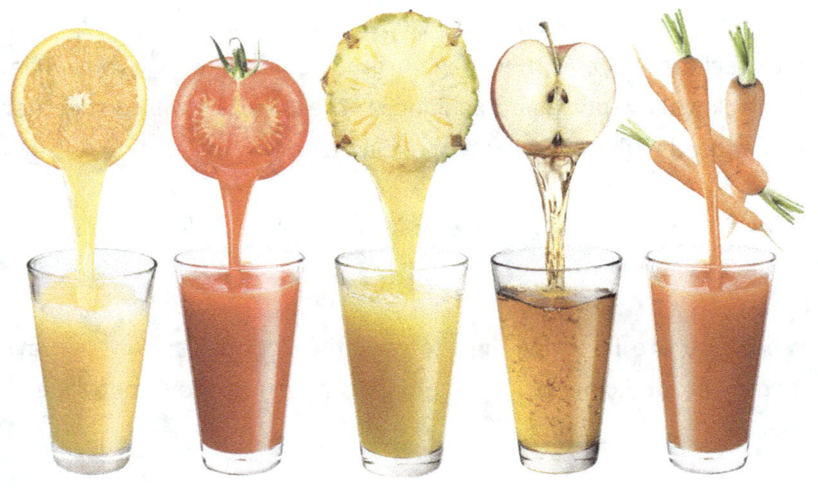

Natural Fruit Juice

One simple yet effective strategy is to use natural fruit juices as a way to alleviate the presence of external cysts and painful blackheads.

You use these juices as a topical application, stirring a bit of cucumber or citric fruit juice with a bit of almond oil.

Once mixed up, apply it the entire area where acne exists and leave on for a period of 15 minutes. Rinse off with lukewarm water and pat dry.

Almond oil and other natural substances like it, are easy remedies that will help remove acne if applied regularly.

Do this 2-3 times each week.

You can also replace cucumber juice with apricot juice or lemon juice, as long as they are natural with no added sweeteners or sugars.

Fenugreeks Leaf Remedy

Rather than cure acne, fenugreek leaves help prevent acne from returning once you have it under control. You simply crush the leaves into a small bowl, and add water to form a paste.

Apply this to your face, as a mask, and leave it on overnight. Make sure to use an old pillowcase, as it can leave light stains.

Mask Of Honey

Honey contains natural antibacterial qualities and is often used as a facemask in spas and home treatments. These masks are inexpensive and can be purchased from your local drug store.

Apply the mask once or twice a week, and enjoy the results. It works exceptionally well!

White Vinegar Treatment

Once again, this is a topical treatment that works wonders. With a cotton ball, soak in white vinegar and apply to infected area, leaving it on for 5-15 minutes.

Rinse off with cold water. If you find the vinegar too strong, dilute it with 1/3 cup of water, and apply.

Oatmeal Mask

Simply cook a small amount of plain oatmeal and apply to your face. Allow this mixture to set on your face for 15 minutes before rinsing off.

Oatmeal acts as a natural exfoliate, and provides instant relief. Try to integrate this method at least twice a week, as it takes very little time and effort and will yield great results.

Yeast Solution

Mix 1 tablespoon of dried or fresh yeast with 2 tablespoons of lemon juice; apply on face, wait until it gets hard (try not to move), peel or wash with warm water.

Bay Leaf Remedy

Grind bay leaves and blanch in warm water, Cool and apply to your face. Rinse off after ten minutes.

Lettuce Solution

Saturate clean, rinsed lettuce leaves in water. Rinse your face with the water.

Tea Bag Cure

Mix 2-3 tea bags to some basil and cook in boiling water for 10-20 minutes. Then apply on the acne with a clean cotton ball.

The home remedies listed above are ones that been used over the years successfully.

Personally, I have found the honey mask to work wonders, and the Oatmeal mask formula has helped me keep my acne under control without the need for expensive third party treatments.

Chapter 5- Proven Methods Of Treating Acne

Being that skin conditions differ in so many ways (oily, normal, dry, or combination skin) there is no such thing as a one-size-fits-all acne cure.

Recently, the FDA has sanctioned the use of a gel called Epiduo for acne-affected patients over the age of 12 years.

Prescribed for a one-time use on a daily basis, Epiduo is a combination of two time-tested treatments for acne. Benzoyl peroxide 2.5% and Adapalene 0.1% contained in Epiduo are generically sold and goes by the name Differin.

The manufacturers of Epiduo, Galderma had stated in a recent press release that the Epiduo gel has been able to combine the two for the first time and it would hit the market early 2009.

Several other over-the-counter medications such as Stri-dex, Clearsil, Clearstick and Oxy Night Watch contain a key acne fighting ingredient; Salicylic Acid.

If the acne is very severe and a cyst has formed making other medications immune, then a potent Retinoid called Isotretinoin can be used orally.

Oral antibiotics have also become commonly used in order to keep acne breakouts at bay. The antibiotics help to subside the inflammation with initial high doses that are later cut down gradually. But if the acne becomes resistant to the antibiotic over time, it cannot be controlled.

In the US, many broad-spectrum antibiotics have been in use for the purpose of treating acne.

A visit to a dermatologist for a detailed examination is the best way to find out the treatment that will work for you.

Your dermatologist will be able to determine the best treatment for you depending on the condition of your acne as well as your personal skin type.

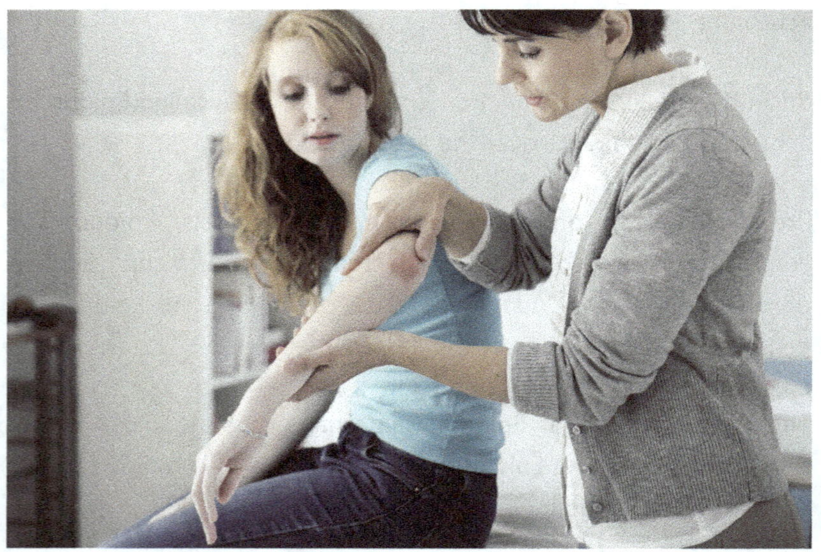

CHAPTER 6- HOME TREATMENTS & REMEDIES

If you're willing to walk on the wild side and risk the strange, inquisitive looks from friends and family members who might catch you in the act, here are my personal favorite home based acne remedies ;)

NOTE: All of these remedies are entirely safe.

Toothpaste Solution

When I first heard about this home based remedy, I'll be honest, I thought there was no way in heck this was going to work. Still, with nothing to lose, I decided to give it a shot and was very glad I did.

Not only does it work exceptionally well, but also takes only a few seconds to do.

All you need is a dab of your favorite toothpaste.

Apply a small amount to your acne spots, zores and zits and leave it on to dry overnight. (Make sure to use an old pillowcase).

You can also substitute toothpaste with baking soda and water.

Rinse it off in the morning, and you're done! Do this 2-3 times a week during painful breakouts

Aspirin Mask

Dermatologists have approved aspirin as a way of developing a facemask to help combat acne. This is a safe and effective method and not only does it have the potential to relieve acne, but it can also help to minimize existing scars!

Here is how you create your aspirin mask:

Supplies:

- Honey
- Non coated aspirin (any brand)
- Neutrogena Healthy Skin Anti-Wrinkle Cream
- Alcohol Free Skin Toner

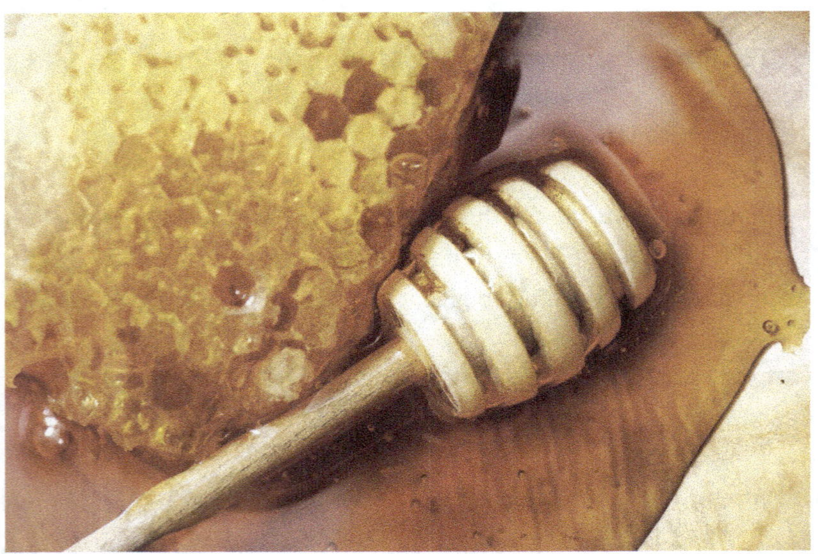

Recipe:

1) Take four aspirin tablets and place them into a small bowl.

2) Sprinkle water onto the aspirin. Do NOT use too much water, or the aspirin will dissolve, just sprinkle a few drops to loosen it up. Using your fingers rub the water and aspirin together to blend it well and break the tablets apart.

The texture of your mix should be very grainy.

3) Now, add two teaspoons of honey to your mixture. Mix the formula together well, so that the aspirin, water and honey are thoroughly blended.

4) Apply the mixture to your face making sure to avoid getting any into your eyes. Once you have your face entirely covered with the aspirin mask, leave it on for ten minutes.

Do not touch it or rub it in once it's on your face. After the ten minutes are up, rinse the formula from you face with cool water, which rubbing the grains of aspirin all over your face (exfoliating your skin).

5) Next, after washing it from your skin, use the toner to blot your face, smoothing it all over. This will also remove any excess formula and leave your face feeling brand new.

6) And finally, use the moisturizer that you purchase as a final touch to polish up your face and replace the moisture. Your moisturizer should contain retinol, which will tighten up your face and reduce the appearance of wrinkles and lines.

Repeat 2-3 times a week.

Ice, Ice Baby

Another easy home based remedy that worked wonders each time I used this method during extreme breakouts. All you have to do is apply a cold compact (or bag of broken ice) to your face every night before bed.

A wet towel will also work well, as it will reduce swelling and help to eliminate clogged pores that cause breakouts.

Milk Of Magnesia (Three Part Process)

This is a great home based cleanser that is absolutely safe to use. Simply apply it to the infected area and leave on for 10-15 minutes before rinsing off.

Then, dissolve one teaspoon of Epsom salt (Magnesium Sulphate) into a 3/4 of hot water.

Apply to the infected area with a clean cloth (avoid cotton balls as they may stick to the skin and cause blocked pores). Leave on for 20 minutes before rinsing off with cold water.

Finally, the third part involves creating a home-based toner. You simply add 3 drops of Benzoin oil or peroxide into a cup of cold water.

Wash down your face with this solution and rinse off.

This is an antibacterial remedy, and it works very well, so give it a shot!

Sandalwood Powder

All you need for this remedy is one teaspoon of sandalwood powder and one teaspoon of tumeric.

Mix this with a small amount of white milk (any kind). Spread over infected areas, leaving it on for 15-25 minutes. Rinse off with warm water, and pat dry.

This can take a couple of sessions to begin working but produces incredible results. Once again, it's entirely safe to do as many times as you wish.

The Oiled Up Strategy

This is one of the most effective methods I've ever tried, and it was a regular routine during bouts of extreme acne and flare-ups.

All you need for this acne-free recipe is a small bottle of castor oil, and a small bottle of extra virgin olive oil or Jojoba oil, which works just as well. Virgin oil will provide moisture to your skin and also will draw out any bacteria that may be trapped under the surface of your skin.

Furthermore, virgin oil will also fortify your skin with its natural antioxidants.

Create a mixture consisting of 1/2 olive oil and 1/2 castor oil, equally mixed. You can experiment with other portions later on, but when starting out it's always recommended to begin with an equal half and half mixture.

Once mixed together, gently massage it all over the affected areas of your body (you can use this anywhere you like including your face, neck, upper body and back). Once you have smoothed it over all of your infected areas, lay a warm compact such as a towel or washcloth over the area for 10-15 minutes.

What this does is naturally steams your face which allows your pores to breath and open up, releasing toxins from beneath the surface of your skin.

Leave the solution on your body with the compact serving as a sealant for 10-15 minutes. Then, massage the oils into your skin again before rinsing off with cold water (not warm, as cold will tighten your skin and close your pores).

If you choose to use olive oil make sure that you purchase extra virgin, not.

A Vitamin A Day, Keeps Acne At Bay

Taking a multi-vitamin every day can help control acne, by ensuring that your skin is given proper nutrition and that your body is not producing an abundance of sebum (which is responsible for clogging pores).

Another useful tip is in adding chromium to your diet, a supplement focused on healing skin infections.

CHAPTER 7- ACNE SCARS REMOVAL

If you have been left with excessive scarring caused by acne, there are things you can do to minimize and eliminate scarring.

One of these options is called laser re-surfacing, which is conducted within a hospital or medical center by a doctor or dermatologist, and is a corrective surgical method that will quickly eliminate the appearance of scarring. With this technique, the top layer of your skin is removed, revealing a clean, fresh layer without scars.

This is similar to laser eye surgery, where one thin layer of damaged tissue is removed so that a new, untouched layer is exposed, instantly correcting and removing any scarring or damage.

The only downside to this procedure is the costs involved. Re-surfacing can be very expensive however it is a sure-fire method of permanently removing scarring caused by extreme acne.

For deep acne scars, there is a procedure called the punch graft. This is where good, healthy skin is removed from other parts of the body and used to replace scarred skin by way of grafting.

If you are interested in finding out more about these methods, contact your local dermatologist for a free consultation.

Laser resurfacing is the only definite solution to removing permanent scarring, however there are also home based remedies that will fade scars, but will not entirely remove them.

One of these treatments is completed by rubbing Vitamin E onto your scarred area. You can purchase Vitamin E is liquid form, or as a capsule that you can cut open and extract the vitamin to rub it onto your scarred areas.

You can also try rubbing virgin olive oil onto your scars regularly, which has been said to help reduce the appearance of scars.

Chapter 8 - Medications

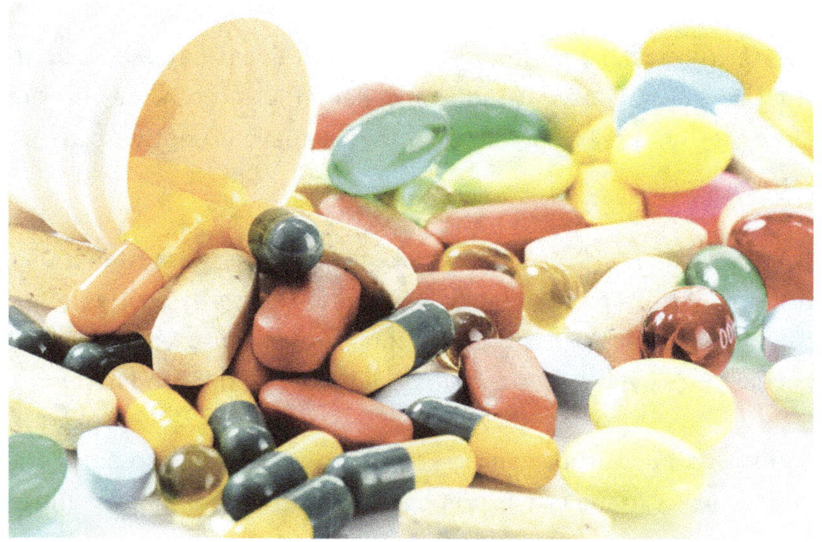

Medication for acne can either be topical or systemic.

Topical medications are to be applied on the skin where as systemic medications are consumed. The main aim of the medications is to remove acne from the roots by curing the factors that lead to the formation of acne.

Here are some medicines that are used to treat acne.

Oral antibiotics are often used to cure acne. This is usually administered to people who suffer from acne consistently.

However the bacteria that causes acne can soon become impervious to the antibiotics and thus refuse to treat the acne. The doctors then will generally prescribe a different round of antibiotics to help the cause. The most common kinds of antibiotics used are erythromycin and tertracycline and its derivatives.

However, erythromycin leads to discomfort in the gastrointestinal tract and tetracycline and its derivatives are not suitable for pregnant women and children who are not yet eight years old. The components of these antibiotics heal the pustule or swelling by drying them up internally.

Topical retinoids is another set of medications that are used to treat acne. They are derived from Vitamin A and can prevent the closing of the pores. By doing so they actually do not let acne be formed.

They include gels or creams like adapalene, tazarotene and tretinoin. The topical retinoids can cause rashes as well as other such irritations. They can cause sunburns because your skin will become more vulnerable to UV rays when using this product.

You would need to use sunscreen if you apply these creams. It is important to contact your skin specialist before you opt for these medications.

Corticosteroid injections are given to patients with acne only when the acne has swelled to an extent of bursting. Thus the swelling diminishes and the acne dries up at a faster rate.

For cystic acne and severe cases of acne, isoretinoin is used. This is only for extreme cases and for healing intricate acne problems.

Oral contraceptives are effective medications for healing acne but also have their limitations. They are not meant for women smokers, women above 35 years of age, or for women who suffer from problems relating to blood clotting.

Oral contraceptives diminish the excess secretion from the glands and thus regulate the hormones to control acne.

 Tropical antimicrobials are used to treat moderated acne problems. These medications attack the bacterial colonies.

These medications can be taken individually or coupled with others that treat certain causes for acne formation. They include azelaic acid, benzoyl peroxide, clindamycin, erythromycin and sodium sulfacetamide. Where as azelaic acid and clindamycin lessen the bacterial growth, benzoyl peroxide kills the bacteria to treat acne.

A blend of erythromycin with benzoyl peroxide is extremely proficient in treating acne. However, these medications have certain adverse effects.

CHAPTER 9- HORMONAL TREATMENTS

Hormones play a very significant role in acne formation. The male hormone, androgen, as well as the female hormone, estrogen, contribute to acne formation.

These hormones are released during puberty and also during menstruation and pregnancy. This is why a larger percentage of females in comparison to males suffer from acne.

A proper hormone balance can be achieved by several methods. These include healthy eating habits, getting rid of strain, taking in a lot of water, and also regularly exercising.

These excess harmful toxins as well as the hormones need to be excreted from your system. This is generally carried out by the kidneys and liver.

However what you need to understand is that these organs cannot function effectively if you have an unhealthy diet. You should consume a well-balanced meal so that your body receives all the necessary nutrients and can work proficiently.

Too much of any constituent will ultimately lead to a loss of another and harm your body's system. This will consequently damage your skin.

The natural treatments include the use of antioxidants that balance the hormones and also clean the blood so that it is free of harmful toxins.

Additionally, try to drink a lot of water and keep away from coffee can keep acne outbreaks at bay. Avoid stress and anxiety, exercise regularly, and keep away from oily foods. All of these measures tend to restrict the release of excess hormones and prevent acne formation.

Corticosteroids are effective in reducing blemishes. But excess of such medicine can also be harmful - that is why you should always consult your physician before you choose to take them.

The best way to balance hormones is through natural processes. They guarantee great results and carry with them, no risks of side effects.

Chapter 10- The Acne Free System

For those who have acne, it is a very good idea to have a diet that contains an abundance of fresh fruits and vegetables. Also, make it a point to drink a lot of water regularly to keep your system flushed out and toxins consistently removed from your system. Eight to ten glasses a day will suffice.

Another good idea is to focus on incorporating a diet rich with antioxidants and fiber.

These are ingredients in the diet that will keep your skin healthy and fit and enable you to look good and feel great.

Another thing considered to be very good for fighting acne is protein. Vitamin A is also considered by health experts to be a great weapon against acne.

Oregon Grape And Echinacea

These are two herbs that are exceptional at boosting your body's immune system and will also help minimize bacteria known to trigger or cause acne flare-ups.

In order to consistently manage and eliminate acne, you need to develop a system that involves a good diet as well as following a regimen that incorporates acne-fighting elements into your daily life.

Do not deviate from this system until your acne is well under control. It takes time and effort to combat acne, but if you follow the strategies featured within this guide, you will be well on your way to permanently eliminating acne from your life.

You deserve to look and feel your best. By researching your options, consulting with a skin care specialist and implementing small changes to your diet and surroundings, you can get acne under control once and for all.

To living acne free!

ABOUT THE AUTHOR

Heather Rose is a health specialist. She aims to improve the health of individuals both physical and mental. She works daily with people who have mental problems and some of them have self-esteem issues because of physical ailments.

Heather loves people and helping them brings her joy. She has written many books that aims to help people address issues in their lives and how to deal with people with special needs.

She writes from years of experience and her writings are very easy to read, practical and effective.

www.ingramcontent.com/pod-product-compliance
Lightning Source LLC
Chambersburg PA
CBHW070100260726

48658CB00002B/920